M000302066

How To Support Children
with Problem Behavior

PRO-ED Series on Autism Spectrum Disorders
Edited by Richard L. Simpson

Titles in the Series

PRO-ED Series on Autism Spectrum Disorders

HOW TO SUPPORT CHILDREN WITH PROBLEM BEHAVIOR

Stephen C. Luce and Angela F. Smith

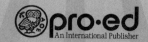

An International Publisher

8700 Shoal Creek Boulevard
Austin, Texas 78757-6897
800/897-3202   Fax 800/397-7633
www.proedinc.com

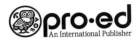

© 2007 by PRO-ED, Inc.
8700 Shoal Creek Boulevard
Austin, Texas 78757-6897
800/897-3202   Fax 800/397-7633
www.proedinc.com

Library of Congress Cataloging-in-Publication Data

Luce, Stephen C.
   How to support children with problem behavior / Stephen C. Luce and Angela F.
Smith; edited by Richard L. Simpson.
      p. cm.
   Includes bibliographical references.
   ISBN-13: 978-1-4164-0148-3
   ISBN-10: 1-4164-0148-2 (softcover : alk. paper)
   1. Behavior disorders in children—Treatment.   2. Problem children—Behavior
modification.   3. Problem children—Education.   I. Smith, Angela F.   II. Title.
RJ506.B44L78   2007
618.92'8914—dc22

                                                                    2005035705

Art Director: Jason Crosier
Designer: Nancy McKinney
This book is designed in Nexus Serif TF and Neutra Text.

Printed in the United States of America

4   5   6   7   8   9   10   11   23   22   21   20   19   18   17   16

Contents

About Autism Spectrum Disorders

Autism spectrum disorders (ASD) are complex, neurologically based developmental disabilities that typically appear early in life. The Autism Society of America (2004) estimates that as many as 1.5 million people in the United States have autism or some form of pervasive developmental disorder. Indeed, its prevalence makes ASD an increasingly common and currently the fastest growing developmental disability. ASD are perplexing and enigmatic. According to the *Diagnostic and Statistical Manual of Mental Disorders,* individuals with ASD have difficulty in interacting normally with others; exhibit speech, language, and communication difficulties (e.g., delayed speech, echolalia); insist on routines and environmental uniformity; engage in self-stimulatory and stereotypic behaviors; and respond atypically to sensory stimuli (American Psychiatric Association, 2000; Simpson & Myles, 1998). In some cases, aggressive and self-injurious behavior may be present in these individuals. Yet, in tandem with these characteristics, children with ASD often have normal patterns of physical growth and development, a wide range of cognitive and language capabilities, and some individuals with ASD have highly developed and unique abilities (Klin, Volkmar, & Sparrow, 2000). These widely varied characteristics necessitate specially designed interventions and strategies orchestrated by knowledgeable and skilled professionals.

Preface to the Series

Teaching and managing learners with ASD can be demanding, but favorable outcomes for children and youth with autism and autism-related disabilities depend on professionals using appropriate and valid methods in their education. Because identifying and correctly using effective teaching methods is often enormously challenging (National Research Council, 2001; Simpson et al., 2005), it is the intent of this series to provide professionals with scientifically based methods for intervention. Each book in the series is designed to assist professionals and parents in choosing and correctly using a variety of interventions that have the potential to produce significant benefits for children and youth with ASD. Written in a user-friendly, straightforward fashion by qualified and experienced professionals, the books are aimed at individuals who seek practical solutions and strategies for successfully working with learners with ASD.

Richard L. Simpson
Series Editor

References

American Psychiatric Association. (2000). *Diagnostic and statistical manual of mental disorders* (4th ed., text rev.). Washington, DC: Author.

Autism Society of America. (2004). *What is autism?* Retrieved March 11, 2005, from http://autism-society.org

Klin, A., Volkmar, F., & Sparrow, S. (2000). *Asperger syndrome.* New York: Guilford Press.

National Research Council. (2001). *Educating children with autism.* Committee on Educational Interventions for Children with Autism, Division of Behavioral and Social Sciences and Education. Washington, DC: National Academy Press.

Simpson, R., de Boer-Ott, S., Griswold, D., Myles, B., Byrd, S., Ganz, J., et al. (2005). *Autism spectrum disorders: Interventions and treatments for children and youth.* Thousand Oaks, CA: Corwin Press.

Simpson, R. L., & Myles, B. S. (1998). *Educating children and youth with autism: Strategies for effective practice.* Austin, TX: PRO-ED.

Introduction to Applied Behavior Analysis

For a variety of reasons, behavior patterns develop differently in children, and the development can be more variable in children with disabilities like autism and other developmental disorders involving abnormal neurological development. Some behaviors are more troublesome than others, and we will be discussing behaviors that may need to be reduced. The significance of a behavior depends on the circumstances and the needs of the individual. Some behaviors may be significant because of the potential for harm to the individual, as in the case of self-injurious behavior. Other behaviors may be serious impediments to the child's development, as in the case of poor hygiene or social skills. What is a significant behavior problem for some may not be for others. For example, excessively eating sweets may have mild health implications for some children, but for a child with diabetes or morbid obesity, it becomes serious.

This manual, which is an update of one done earlier (Luce & Christian, 1981), is designed to provide caregivers with information that will be useful in the design of procedures to support children with behavior problems. The information is based on research conducted over the last 50 years that has been validated in schools, homes, and other community settings with children exhibiting behavior disorders (Bailey & Burch, 2002; Sidman, 1966). For additional information about empirically validated procedures with this population, see Lovaas (2003) and Maurice, Green, and Luce (1996). This particular manual is devoted to the needs of children with autism spectrum disorders; however, treatment methods similar to those described here have been shown to be effective with children with other developmental disabilities, as well as with acquired disorders such as traumatic brain injury.

To clarify the concepts and techniques presented in this manual, we have included multiple examples encountered in our extensive clinical practice over the years. Once concepts have been introduced and illustrated with real examples (the names used are fictitious), exercises are provided to help the reader practice the terminology and plan interventions with individuals in their lives who need support for behavior disorders or problems. It is important for the reader to work through the exercises, as they are designed to improve learning through active involvement with the concepts presented.

Although the concepts described in this book have been derived from the professional scientific literature, we have attempted to minimize the use of technical language in hopes of conveying the salient points without requiring the reader to spend time learning new definitions. The recommendations made in this manual are based on extensive research conducted in hundreds of clinical settings by thousands of distinguished clinicians (Cooper, Heron, & Heward, 1987; Miltenberger, 2001; Sulzer-Azaroff & Mayer, 1991). We are very grateful to our colleagues for developing such effective procedures to address problem behaviors with children.

Some readers will use this manual in association with a college or graduate school course about behavior. Others may read the material with the support of one or more people who have practiced the procedures on their own. Support of a knowledgeable person is always advised because some of the techniques presented have subtle characteristics that may not be fully exposed in this short manual. The following scenario provides an example of a professional and a parent working together:

> Mrs. Frederick was the mother of a 6-year-old boy with autism. Over the years, Larry, her son, began to exhibit behaviors that his parents and teachers referred to as "difficulty with transitions." He would get so involved in his activity that changing to another activity was met with great resistance. On some occasions, he would react to changes so strongly that he would strike out at his teachers or parents rather than proceed to the next activity. When confronted with an unanticipated change in activities, he would sometimes throw a large tantrum. For example, when his school had to be closed at noon because of a snowstorm, he was distressed for hours after safely reaching home on the school bus. Mrs. Frederick consulted with Larry's teacher, who had developed a program for Larry at school. The prescribed program was difficult for his mom to understand. For example, even though Larry was in obvious distress during these episodes associated with changes in routine, his teacher was advising that his behavior be ignored. That did not seem right to Mrs. Frederick. Larry's teacher gave Mrs. Frederick some written material describing effective behavioral procedures. After a week of reading, Mrs. Frederick and Larry's teacher met again to discuss the procedure being used at school. Mrs. Frederick began to understand the rationale for ignoring the behavior and recognized that Larry's program included close supervision to ensure that he would not hurt himself or anyone around him. He was given loving attention when he was able to calm down or when he tolerated the changes in routine. It also became apparent to Mrs. Frederick that for Larry to fully benefit from the teaching procedures, they should be carried out at home as well as at school.

In this example, Mrs. Frederick gained access to material like that contained in this manual through her son's teacher. Often parents discover the manual or similar material on their own. To get support for implementation of the procedures outlined in this manual, parents may seek the advice of school personnel, psychologists in the community, or other parents who have discovered the utility of behavioral procedures.

As was previously mentioned, the procedures outlined in this manual have been closely scrutinized in scientific journals devoted to the education and support of people with challenging behavior. The technical name for the procedures used to test and validate the procedures described is *applied behavior analysis*. In some circles, these procedures may be described within the context of *positive behavior support* or *learning theory*. The key element of all the procedures is their proven track record. They have been carefully analyzed and shown to be effective in children with behavior problems (Baer, Wolf, & Risley, 1968). The following scenario illustrates how commonly used support strategies are sometimes introduced in a manner that does not allow us to analyze their effects on behavior:

> Hannah was a 5-year-old girl with some learning disabilities who had a difficult time engaging in quiet activities in preschool and at home. Because she was going to start kindergarten in the autumn, Hannah's mom consulted their pediatrician about her activity level, and the doctor prescribed a medication designed to slow Hannah down at school.
>
> Hannah's mom was delighted to hear that Hannah's performance at school was good, and her teacher reported that she adjusted well to kindergarten. Hannah's mother attributed her daughter's success at school to the medication prescribed by the pediatrician. Hannah's teacher assumed the success at school was the result of the structure at school, such as rules and schedules designed to be balanced and interesting to the students, as well as other tricks she had learned in her 10 years of teaching kindergarten.

Generally, when trying to determine the effects of a behavioral intervention, it is recommended that one intervention be introduced at a time. In the preceding example, it would be difficult to determine whether Hannah's medication or the structure of the classroom helped her to perform well. In the case of medical interventions for behavior, such as the prescription used with Hannah, it may be desirable to minimize the risk of adverse side effects associated with the medication by *withdrawing* the medication after a few weeks at school to determine if it was necessary. If, after Hannah received no medication, her behavior deteriorated, one could support the use of the medication in the future, assuming there were no hidden risks associated with it. If the medication was withdrawn and Hannah remained productive and well behaved, we would never know if it had any positive effects on her, but we would be justified in keeping her off the medication in the future. Systematic changes in a child's environment or how we interact with them

3

can lead us to important information about what works and does not work for an individual child. Mrs. Washington changed her teaching methods systematically in the following scenario:

> Mrs. Washington was a third-grade teacher who was concerned about the spelling performance of her students. Ten new spelling words were presented each week, and the words were used in stories and exercises each day throughout the week. Each Friday afternoon, there was a spelling test in which Mrs. Washington read out the words and asked each student to write the word on a piece of paper. During the months of September and October, the students averaged only 60% correct spelling words.
>
> Using the spelling test scores over the first 8 weeks of school as a *baseline,* Mrs. Washington graphed the average performance of her students and saw no improvement over the period. In November, she started to provide time each day for the students to write the words in sentences. In addition, on two to three occasions each week, she instituted a game involving children doing time trials on a computer to see how fast they could spell out five of the week's spelling words. The implementation of those extra exercises reduced spelling errors on the weekly tests dramatically throughout November, December, and for 2 weeks in January. Mrs. Washington thought it might be time to stop the exercises in January and February, only to find that the spelling scores began to slip again. In March she reinstituted the exercises, and the spelling errors were again reduced.

Mrs. Washington implemented a series of extra exercises each week after a period of time without the exercises. That period before the extra exercises were implemented is called the *baseline.* When she implemented the exercises, she could measure subsequent performance on the spelling tests against that baseline. After several weeks with the extra exercises, she removed them, only to see the spelling scores deteriorate. When the extra spelling exercises were reinstituted, the spelling scores again improved. Figure 1 shows the way it looks when graphed.

By starting the extra exercises after a baseline was established and later withdrawing them for a few weeks, Mrs. Washington made it clear that her implementation of extra exercises was responsible for the improvement in spelling scores. The fact that the students' performance improved during both periods of time when the extra exercises were in place and deteriorated when they were not part of the classroom routine provides us with clear evidence of the effects of her treatment procedure. We call that a *withdrawal, reversal,* or *ABAB design,* where condition A was without extra exercises and condition B was with them.

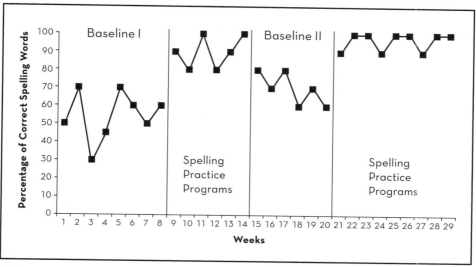

FIGURE 1. The average number of words correctly spelled by students in Mrs. Washington's third-grade classroom. During baseline, 10 spelling words were presented each week and tested on Friday afternoon. During special practice programs, Mrs. Washington provided practice sessions each day, as well as spelling games two or three times per week. The spelling practice programs improved student performance over the weeks in which practice sessions were not provided.

The following scenario illustrates another method of analyzing behavior:

Jimmy was a 7-year-old boy with Down syndrome and pervasive developmental disorders who had trouble sharing in the classroom and at home. During free time at school, the students in Jimmy's class were allowed to go to the activities centers in the classroom to engage in a number of play and learning experiences. There was a kitchen area with child-sized kitchen appliances, there was a Lego center for building things, and there was a quiet reading center. Jimmy usually migrated to the kitchen center, and if another child was playing with a pan or utensil that attracted him, he found it difficult to refrain from grabbing the object out of the hands of his classmate. When his classmates resisted, Jimmy sometimes became very angry and threw a temper tantrum that was disruptive to his classroom and unpleasant for the other students.

Jimmy's teacher recognized that sharing was an important behavior for him to learn to help him decrease the number of disruptive behaviors exhibited during playtime. She noticed similar sharing problems when Jimmy was on the playground, and in speaking to his mother, she discovered that he also had difficulty sharing with his three brothers and sisters.

Jimmy's teacher decided to set up a token system for him. She carefully counted his tantrums during playtime and on the playground, and she explained the counting system to Jimmy's mom, who was then able to count the behaviors at home. Jimmy's teacher explained to him that for every minute that he was able to play nicely and share the toys, he would get a star on his chart. When he received 10 stars, he could have access to some new toys that had arrived from the supply store recently and had not yet been put in their respective areas. The play sessions were 15 minutes in length, making it possible for Jimmy to play nicely for 10 minutes and then gain access to special toys for the 5 remaining minutes of the play session.

During the morning and afternoon play sessions in the classroom, Jimmy's performance improved dramatically with the new system. After a week of successful playtime in the classroom with only a few sharing problems, Jimmy's teacher implemented the token system on the playground as well. Jimmy's parents and teacher were very interested to note that each time the token system was implemented in a new setting, the behaviors there improved. Improvement was even noted at home when his parents arranged a similar program to encourage good sharing and fewer tantrums.

Improvement in Jimmy's behavior coincided with the implementation of the star token system. Improvement was seen first in the indoor play areas, then on the playground, and finally at home at the same time the tokens were introduced. This demonstration of effectiveness in three different settings (called a "multiple baseline") is the level of proof we would like to have to speak confidently about a procedure.

Figure 2 depicts the data compiled on Jimmy. Jimmy's teacher used an interval measure in which she recorded each minute, whether or not Jimmy exhibited any disruptive behavior during the minute. She chose to graph the number of minutes *without* disruption, so high numbers in Figure 2 indicate low disruptions. The top graph shows the number of disruptions in the morning play session, the second shows the disruptions during the afternoon play session on the playground, and the third shows the disruptions at home during a play session of equal duration. In each case, the data before the dashed line represent the baseline, and the data after the dashed line represent Jimmy's behavior after the token system was implemented. Because the token system was implemented first in the morning session and subsequently in the other sessions, and the behavior improved only when the token system was implemented, we have good evidence that the token system caused the change in behavior. Without such a systematic demonstration of

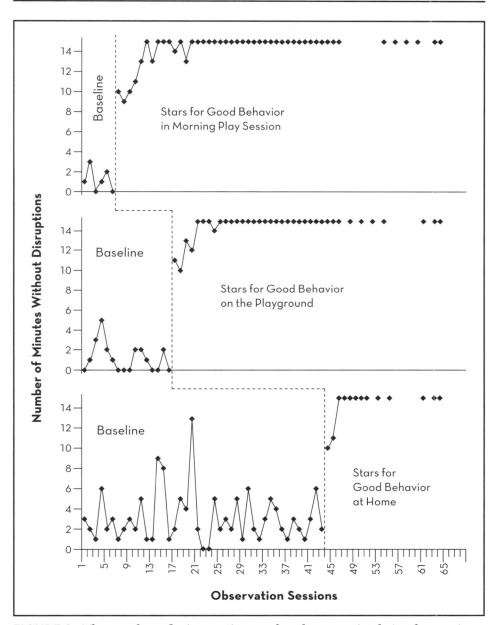

FIGURE 2. The number of minutes Jimmy played appropriately in play sessions held in the classroom, on the school playground, and at home. During baseline, Jimmy's disruptive behavior and appropriate play were ignored. During treatment, a star system was used to reinforce Jimmy for not exhibiting disruptive behaviors. The star system was introduced sequentially in each setting, proving a multiple-baseline verification of the effects of the star system.

effectiveness, we might occasionally attribute success to procedures that are ineffective or pass up a procedure that seemed ineffective.

EXERCISES

Practice what you have learned about describing and analyzing behavior by answering the following questions:

1. Describe an event in your child's life that you think is having an effect on his or her behavior. How could you convert that positive or negative event into a procedure to change your child's behavior?
2. Can you think of a way to systematically introduce that procedure to validate its effectiveness?
3. Many people think sugar affects children. Some say that when their children eat sweet food, they become more active. How could you test the effects of sweet food on your child? Draw a picture of an imaginary graph that shows the use of a reversal design to analyze the effects of sugar in a child's breakfast and its effects on disciplinary problems at school or home.

Identifying Behaviors in Need of Reduction

Some of the behaviors we select for reduction are behaviors that cause injury; other behaviors may be selected that, if exhibited in the community, may be stigmatizing for the child or disturbing to the general public. Under any of those circumstances, those responsible for the child may decide to work on decreasing the impact of the behavior. Most behaviors in need of reduction are selected because they meet the definition of a problem behavior. By *problem behavior* we mean behavior that without reduction will limit the child's potential to develop skills, live at home, and attend school without continued intensive support. The following examples depict behaviors that parents, teachers, and other interested persons have selected for reduction. These are behaviors that may be exhibited too frequently for the children to progress satisfactorily and gain the full benefits of their lives in the community:

Self-Injurious Behavior

Billy was a 13-year-old who never learned to talk but seemed to understand much of what was said to him. At times, he would hit his head with his hands. This was especially a problem in school and seemed to occur when he was asked to do an assignment or task. The problem became so serious that the teachers in his classroom were reluctant to make requests of Billy for fear that he might hurt himself. Billy's doctor noted that his ears and eyes were bruised and swollen from the hitting and warned his parents that continued self-injury of that intensity could result in problems with his vision. The behavior was affecting his health and his education.

Disruptive Behavior

Lisa was an active 10-year-old who could make single-word requests but primarily echoed the language of others around her. Several times a day, she exhibited severe temper tantrums during which she sometimes caused property destruction. For example, one day at school she became very upset and threw some furniture, causing a chair to go through a large window in the classroom. When her teachers tried to contain her, she would become very threatening, and, although it had never happened before, she injured two of her teachers in the same week. Concerns for the safety of her peers as well as the teachers and Lisa herself caused the school principal to recommend a transfer for Lisa to another school in a different part of the school district.

Self-Stimulatory Behavior

Henry was a very happy 4-year-old child with autism who spent a great deal of time waving his hands in front of his face. When he was left alone, he typically went to a corner of the room and shook his fingers in front of his eyes, while looking through them at light sources. His parents reported that when he engaged in this behavior, it was difficult to get his attention and that, in some instances, in the community, people would stare, make comments, or even tease Henry.

In the past, we often referred to behaviors that we target to reduce as *maladaptive* or *dysfunctional*. Some behavior analysts still use those terms, but if we consider what controls the problem behavior, we often discover that the behavior is adaptive and serves a distinct function for the child. The case of Emily provides an example of this:

Emily is a precocious 5-year-old who has thrived in both preschool and kindergarten. Because she attends afternoon kindergarten, she is able to stay up later than her sisters did when they were her age. One of her parents usually plays a game of her choice with her after she has bathed and dressed for bed. She loves the special game time that precedes bedtime, and being rather competitive, she often gets very excited when the game "heats up" before going upstairs to bed.

Before first grade and a full day at school commences, her parents realize that she will have to start going to bed earlier, because she will not have the luxury of being able to sleep so late in the mornings when school starts at 8:00 A.M. Her parents tell her that they are going to start moving bedtime to an earlier time to prepare for the new school year, but it becomes difficult to accomplish the earlier bedtime. Emily always seems to have another request for water, a nightlight, her favorite doll, or any number of other things.

Emily begins crying and getting very angry during the bedtime routine. Her parents are worried. They consult the school psychologist, who asks them to log her behavior each evening, paying special attention to the events that come before the behavior as well as those that come after. When the psychologist reviews the logs, she concludes that Emily has learned to delay her bedtime by increasing requests that involve the attention of one of her parents. For her to succeed in a full day of school this bedtime routine is a problem, but it was a very adaptive way for Emily to gain attention and delay bedtime.

Whether a behavior is adaptive like that exhibited in the example of Emily or genuinely maladaptive, it must be determined to be a *true problem* before an effort is made to reduce it. If the behavior is limiting the child in any way, or would be limiting if it persisted later in life, it may be a problem behavior. A behavior that is disruptive or potentially dangerous to the child or others in his environment would be deemed a problem behavior in need of reduction without question.

If adults are considering whether a behavior is truly a problem and worthy of active procedures to reduce it, care is needed. The decision to actively reduce a behavior should be made only when the child and her guardians and caretakers (e.g., teachers and support adults) agree that the behavior is truly a problem for the child. This is usually accomplished with a written plan of treatment that carefully defines the behavior, identifies its problematic qualities, and specifies the procedures that will be used to reduce it. Consider the following scenario in which George's treatment team determines how to address his behaviors:

> George is a 4-year-old boy recently diagnosed with autism. His parents sought and received his admission into a program that provides intensive behavioral intervention for children with autism. In the early stages of training, it became apparent that George engaged in a number of self-stimulatory behaviors that could be considered problem behaviors, as they would draw negative attention in a setting with typically developing children. In addition, the behaviors, which often involve rubbing his face and eyes, disrupt his training exercises.
>
> George's father remembers seeing videotape about early intervention with children like George when he was in college. Understanding that George's behavior can be a problem, he asks the treatment team supervisor if they should be doing something to discourage the self-stimulatory behavior when it is exhibited.
>
> The treatment team determines that a number of the behaviors they are working on, such as eye contact, responding to requests, and imitation, are incompatible with George's self-stimulatory behavior. For example, in order to make eye contact, respond to requests, or imitate motor movements such as "hands up," he will not be able to continue rubbing his face. Therefore, they hold off on reacting to the self-stimulatory behaviors to see if they become less frequent as a result of his improved skills in early training.

In George's case, even though a behavior is potentially a problem behavior, the team decides not to actively set out to reduce it because they hope

11

that with the acquisition of new behaviors such as good attention to task and imitation, the self-stimulatory behaviors will decrease.

EXERCISES

Practice what you have learned about selecting behaviors that are truly a problem by answering the questions below:

1. Make a table listing the problem behaviors exhibited by a child with whom you are working and provide a rationale for actively reducing those behaviors. List any reasons the behaviors limit the child's opportunities, are dangerous to the child or others, or prevent the child from gaining more independence.
2. List all of the people who would need to help the child reduce the behavior. Consider that the most successful procedures used to reduce behavior are carried out in all settings by all those who care for a child.

What Controls Problem Behaviors?

Now that we know how to identify true problem behaviors, we should consider what might be controlling those behaviors when they are exhibited. Most behaviors of concern in children are behaviors that are influenced and controlled by events that occur before and after them. Those controlling variables often reveal the *function* of a behavior. For example, in the case of Emily's behavior before going to bed, her psychologist presumed that the function of her behaviors was to delay her bedtime. It is best to identify the maintaining function of the behavior, or why the behavior is occurring, before choosing a procedure to reduce it. Implementing function-based treatments will increase the probability that the behavior will decrease more successfully than if less informed attempts at treatment are implemented.

In the following scenario, Brianna's team is trying to determine why she has tantrums during playtime:

> Brianna is a 5-year-old nonverbal child with autism. She attends a half-day program that specializes in teaching social skills and other skills to help her in her daily activities, such as brushing her teeth, eating properly, and going to the restroom independently. Brianna has been successful in this program and has learned many self-care and hygiene skills. She has also been able to sit and manipulate toys in a game with peers for up to 1 minute before getting up and running to get another toy. When she runs for another toy, her teacher assumes that she is bored and is finished with the game. However, Mom requests that Brianna learn to play for longer periods of time with peers so that she can play more successfully at her weekly play dates with a typically developing neighbor child. When the teacher attempts to have Brianna engage in play for longer periods of time, her problem behaviors increase dramatically. She throws her body to the floor and has tantrums when prevented from getting another toy. This is the same behavior that Mom sees during play dates with the neighbor child.

Brianna's tantrum behavior is adaptive in her world because she is then able to access the other toys that she wants when she wants them.

However, the behavior is deemed a problem because, without a reduction of the tantrums, she will not be able to participate in school or community play activities in the future. Brianna's mother and teacher struggle to determine how to decrease the tantrums so that she will be able to play with other children, but they have yet to find a solution. Brianna's mom and teacher assume that Brianna does not like to sit in one place for longer than a minute, but they have overlooked the fact that each time she is prevented access to another, more preferred toy, the tantrums appear.

When attempting to identify why a behavior is occurring or what the maintaining function of a behavior is, there are several possibilities. Some of the prominent functions that maintain behavior include (a) access to attention; (b) access to tangibles or items that the individual wishes to possess, consume, or interact with; (c) escape from demands or requests; and (d) automatic functions (e.g., pain attenuation or sensory input).

When you are taking a baseline, we suggest that you also record the events occurring before and after the problem behavior. This will provide you with a functional assessment that is often useful in identifying why a behavior occurs and determining an appropriate procedure to reduce the behavior.

For example, in Brianna's case, a functional assessment would reveal that her tantrums begin after she has played with one toy for about a minute and then is denied access to a new toy (the antecedent) and are followed by her gaining access to a new toy (a tangible consequence). Armed with that information, her team can consider procedures that would enable her to gain the desired tangible consequence while learning to play with a toy for an extended period of time. For example, it might work to allow Brianna to get a new toy after playing with the previous toy for at least 1 minute. One minute was chosen because during baseline, her average duration playing with a toy or activity was 1 minute. That way, in the first stage of training, she would gain access to the desired new activity approximately half the time she attempted to change activities rather than all the time, as when she was in baseline conditions. Over several trials of that scenario, her teachers and parents could slowly increase the time required for her to play with a toy or engage in an activity before she could access a new toy or activity. That procedure would enable Brianna to get what she wants while learning to stick to an activity or play item for extended periods of time, thus increasing her chances to play with peers. Both Mom and Brianna's teacher would have to implement the procedure to ensure that Brianna could play successfully with her peers both at home and in school. If the teacher implemented the procedure at school, but Mom continued to let Brianna frequently get up and get new toys at home, the likelihood of success would be reduced.

In some cases, a functional assessment shows mixed results:

> Stephanie exhibited the same problems at play dates that Brianna had. She also had a short attention span, and her peers were shown

to be prone to playing without her to stay on a task until it was completed. In Stephanie's case, the baseline data looked very similar to Brianna's, but the functional assessment revealed that Stephanie's consequences were different. That is, after a short time playing, she would seek out the attention of an adult, who would lead her back to her peers. In some cases, the adult would hold Stephanie in her lap for some one-to-one attention. If the adult was otherwise occupied, Stephanie would throw a tantrum, just like Brianna.

Stephanie's team would likely look at her baseline data and determine that her behavior was maintained by adult attention. Using a procedure similar to Brianna's, in which adult attention was withheld until Stephanie had completed a specified period of appropriate play, would probably yield good changes in her behavior.

Functional analysis is a process that extends beyond a functional assessment. In some cases, a behavior analyst may choose to run what is called an "analogue functional analysis," in which the number of problem behaviors (or similar behaviors) is recorded during arranged periods of time when the child is given attention, allowed to escape, or left alone (to determine whether the problem behavior occurs in the absence of another person). These analogue conditions, designed to resemble consequences that occur in a natural environment, are repeated over several sessions until the behavior analyst determines the different levels of the behaviors under each analogue. While it is more difficult to conduct a full functional analysis, the information derived from it is very useful and has been shown to be more precise than that obtained from functional assessments. It is recommended that an experienced professional conduct analogue functional analyses to ensure the integrity of the procedures and the safety of the individual.

EXERCISES

1. List the most prominent functions of problem behaviors. If you are not sure of your answer, review the scenarios of Brianna and Stephanie, as well as the preceding paragraph.
2. Sheri, a 6-year-old child with pervasive developmental delay, begins hitting herself in the ear, is running a low-grade fever, and is not sleeping at night. What could be the maintaining function or the "why" of Sheri's behavior? If you are not sure of the answer, review the section between Brianna's and Stephanie's scenarios.
3. How would you describe a problem behavior? For help with this question, review Chapter 1.
4. True or False: When choosing to treat a problem behavior, it is best to treat it only in the home and not in the school setting. (See the example of Brianna for help.)

As stated previously, the decision to target a problem behavior for reduction is one that must be shared by all those caring for the child. For example, if teachers find that a problem behavior arises at school, the cooperation of the parents will be important in order to have a coordinated support program for the child. The child also must be clear on the behavior of concern. If the child is able to understand a description of the behavior, he or she should be clearly informed of the concern about it.

Step One: Defining the Behavior

We specify the problem behavior by *defining* it. A behavioral definition answers five questions:

1. Who emits the behavior?
2. What is the exact behavior?
3. How is the behavior to be measured?
4. When is the behavior to be measured?
5. Where can the behavior be observed and measured?

Once a behavior has been defined, it is sometimes referred to as a *pinpoint* or *target*. Both terms highlight the precision that is needed to carefully evaluate and change behavior. The following scenario illustrates the importance of defining behavior precisely:

> Mrs. Marsh was very concerned about the reports she was receiving about her 8-year-old son, Jeremy. He always received very high grades, especially in subjects that he liked to study on his own. He could tell you every conceivable detail about any plant, animal, or bird that you could think of. However, his teacher reported that he was very rude to her in school and that she had attempted to discipline him without any positive effects. Mrs. Marsh asked for Jeremy to be evaluated by a psychologist in her community, and he

concluded that Jeremy had very low self-esteem, for which he prescribed weekly psychotherapy sessions and a number of changes to his routine at school and at home. After Mrs. Marsh shared the report with Jeremy's teacher, reports coming from the school were mixed. He had good days and bad days. Although he was promoted to the next grade, Mrs. Marsh was very concerned about Jeremy's behavior and the money she was spending on psychotherapy.

The next year, Mrs. Marsh met his new teacher, and she was a little worried when the teacher said that the reports from the psychologist were not very helpful in her preparation for Jeremy joining her class. Instead, the teacher asked Mrs. Marsh to call her back in a week so she could see if Jeremy exhibited any problems, and then she would formulate a plan.

When Mrs. Marsh called back, Jeremy's new teacher had a number of behaviors identified that, if reduced, would help Jeremy succeed better in the classroom. One behavior was called "calling out" and was defined as any time Jeremy called out without raising his hand and waiting for a response from the teacher. A frequency count of that behavior was taken every school day during science class.

As it turned out, many of the behaviors Jeremy exhibited were attempts to correct the answers given to questions raised by the teacher during topics he was particularly knowledgeable about. Despite the fact that correcting other children met with complaints by the children and correcting the teacher was also clearly unwelcome, Jeremy did not respond to their cues. Once the behavior was clearly defined, it was easier for everyone to work on it.

EXERCISE

Now you can practice defining behaviors. Define Jeremy's "calling out" behavior by answering the five questions of a behavioral definition. If you are unsure of the answers, refer to the five questions listed previously in this chapter.

Once you have a complete definition of the problem behavior, it is wise to test the definition by observing the behavior with another person independently at the same time. To the extent that two independent observers agree on the occurrence of a behavior, a definition is said to be reliable. For example, two observers watch a child learning to walk and count the number of consecutive steps the child takes without falling. One observer counts 18, and the other counts 20. Eighteen divided by 20 yields 90% interobserver agreement, or 90% observer reliability. Scores exceeding 80% are usually considered sufficient. It is important to check interobserver agreement or observer reliability every few days to safeguard against losing sight of the behavior definition.

Step Two: Assessing the Behavior

Baseline measures should be taken for several observation sessions before attempting to reduce a behavior. The baseline may show that the behavior is decreasing to a more desirable level, in which case it may not be necessary to introduce a procedure to further reduce it. On the other hand, the baseline may be stable or increasing over time, suggesting that a reduction strategy is needed. The baseline measures are used as a yardstick against which future changes in the behavior can be compared.

There are several ways to measure behavior. Commonly, behavior can be measured by using tally marks on a piece of paper. For example, ₭ would represent five responses. The observer records how often the behavior occurs with a slash mark. This is an example of a frequency of event recording.

In the following scenario, we see how Jeremy's behavior was defined using frequency of event recording, You can compare this definition to the one you created in the previous exercise. Even if your definition is slightly different, it may be reliable. Measurement reliability is the most important gauge of an adequate definition.

> Jeremy's teacher developed a definition for the behavior that led a psychologist to recommend psychotherapy for low self-esteem. The behavior was defined as any time Jeremy corrected a statement made by another student or a teacher, at school during a science lesson. Jeremy's teacher chose to use an event record of the behavior during each science class. The full definition looked like this:
>
> Who? _Jeremy_
>
> What? _Correcting a statement made by a student or teacher regardless of its accuracy_
>
> How? _Event record_
>
> When? _During each science class_
>
> Where? _In the classroom or science lab_

The teacher recorded 8, 6, 3, 12, and 6 statements of correction made by Jeremy on consecutive school days.

When reviewing the event records taken over the week, Jeremy's teacher noted that on Thursdays the science period was 90 minutes instead of the usual 45 to accommodate time in the laboratory. That would explain why on that day Jeremy exhibited 12 responses, which was considerably higher than on the other 4 days. Jeremy's teacher therefore converted each record into the number of responses per hour. For example, on Monday she recorded 4 responses in 60 minutes, or 4 responses per hour. During the 90-minute science period on Thursday, the event record of 12 was divided by 90, yielding a rate of 0.133 responses per minute. Multiplying 0.133 by 60 minutes gave her a figure of 8 responses per hour. Jeremy's teacher compiled the records from science class into a table to send to his parents:

Number of responses	Length of science class in minutes	Responses per hour
8	60	8
6	60	6
3	60	3
12	90	8
6	60	6
Average rate per hour		6.2

As you can see from the preceding table, frequency counts can yield valuable information. In Jeremy's case, because the time spent doing science classes varied, a conversion of the data from frequency to rate provided us with the best information. An event record may be influenced by the number of opportunities a child has to exhibit a behavior, in which case it may be advisable to record the percentage instead of the number of behaviors, as in the following example:

Elijah's parents were hoping to decrease the number of times they had to ask him to follow an instruction. They recorded the number of requests they made of him during 30-minute periods at home after waking up and before the school bus arrived on school days. They noted the number of those requests that he followed appropriately. They found that the number of requests they made varied, so they divided the number of requests that Elijah followed by the total number of requests made during the observation session. For example, Elijah responded appropriately to 4 out of 12 requests one morning in baseline, and they recorded 33% for that day. Later, after training, they counted 5 out of 6 requests as being responded to appropriately and recorded 83%.

Some behaviors are best measured by recording the amount of time spent engaged in the behavior. This is called a "duration measure" and is useful for behaviors of long duration:

> Abu was a young man who spent a great deal of time crying and whining, especially when engaged in schoolwork that he found difficult or frustrating. His teacher first defined the behavior and then set out to make an event record of crying and whining. It soon became apparent that a frequency count would not reflect the true situation. In one 30-minute observation period, for example, Abu exhibited the defined behavior only once, but he was whining and crying for the entire period. When the teacher switched her recording procedure to one of duration, she was able to record when Abu began to cry and when he was able to get back into the scheduled activity. Those working with Abu hoped that the duration of the behavior would decrease.

Similar to a duration measure is *latency,* a measure that works well if you are concerned with the length of time it takes to complete or start a task. Usually, one's latencies decrease as one masters a task. Elijah's case provides an example:

> While measuring the percentage of requests that Elijah followed during the morning routine, his mother and father also recorded the amount of time that elapsed from the time they woke him up in the morning to the time he was dressed and ready to eat breakfast. Once he began to respond more often to the first request made of him, his morning routine went more rapidly and the latency measures decreased. It made the morning routine much more pleasant and efficient, and Elijah never missed the school bus anymore.

We have found that most of the behaviors we deal with in support of children with behavior problems can be assessed using one of the methods just described. Some additional systems such as *interval* and *time sampling* can be useful as well, although they can yield imprecise records if not carefully designed. Jimmy's program in the Introduction to Applied Behavior Analysis section (see Figure 2) used an interval measure. With the assistance of a behavior analyst familiar with the child, families can employ some of the more complex methods of measurement and some alternatives to those procedures described.

Remember, once you have selected a way to define and measure the behavior of concern and have established that the measure is reliable, you should take some time to record the behavior over daily or more frequent observation periods to establish a baseline. Usually, the characteristics of the behavior guide us in determining how often to run observation sessions. For example, if you are measuring a behavior during meals, there are typically three natural opportunities to do that. Getting ready for bed would probably be observed just once a day, and a given academic skill might be observed several times per day.

EXERCISES

1. Define a problem behavior exhibited by a person you know.
   a. Who is the person? Include the name, age, and relationship you have with the person.
   b. What is the behavior?
   c. How could you record the behavior? (List two options.)
   d. When could you observe the behavior?
   e. Where could you observe and measure the behavior?
2. Is the behavior truly a problem? List how the behavior interferes with the person's learning or adjustment by impeding the person or someone in his or her life from functioning to his or her own or society's benefit. For example, it might limit access to work, leisure, or social opportunities.
3. Who would make up this person's team of concerned individuals? For a child, it would likely be his IEP team. For an adult, it might be his or her guardian, if appointed, or loved ones, roommates, or support staff.
4. Who would measure the behavior and determine whether the measures are reliable? List the name and relationship to the person.
5. Who else would be required to monitor the behavior and support the person changing a behavior?
6. Show your answers to a behavior analyst, classmate, or co-worker. Does that person see any problems with your answers? If not, congratulations. If any problems are found, go back and revise the definition before going on to gather your baseline and develop a plan to change the behavior.

Step Three: Changing the Behavior

There are four general strategies available to reduce behavior:

1. Manipulate the environment or the events that precede the behavior.

2. Introduce reinforcement to reduce the problem behavior.
3. Interrupt the events that are found to maintain the behavior.
4. Introduce events that will discourage the behavior in the future.

Manipulating the Environment or Events Preceding the Behavior

Once you have defined a problem behavior and established a baseline level, you can consider different methods to reduce the behavior. When considering the challenging behaviors that prevent their children from engaging in meaningful lives, anticipating what might lead to those behaviors often becomes second nature to parents and caregivers:

> Four-year-old Patricia often throws a temper tantrum on the floor while holding her ears when the telephone rings in her home. Mom has learned to anticipate this and has adapted her phone with a button that lights up with each incoming call. By silencing the ring, Patricia's mother has prevented some of Patricia's tantrums. Events that precede behaviors are called "antecedents." By changing the bell to a light, Patricia's mom has employed an *antecedent management strategy* to avoid her daughter's tantrums.

The Three-Term Contingency Model

The term *contingency* is often used to describe events that occur before and after a behavior, when they influence the behavior. We usually find that similar or identical events precede a problem behavior and follow it each time it occurs. Those events are called "contingent events." Research has shown that key elements of behavior control are found in the events that come immediately before and after the behavior. We refer to a *three-term contingency* in describing the sequence of *antecedent, behavior,* and *consequence.* When determining how to reduce a problem behavior, we consider manipulating the events that precede the behavior (antecedents) and the events that follow the behavior (consequences). Many of the procedures we describe later in the book involve changing the consequences. In this section, we describe procedures that use antecedents to reduce problem behavior.

EXERCISES

See if you can identify the key events preceding Patricia's behavior.

1. What was the antecedent to Patricia's temper tantrums?
2. What was the antecedent control strategy used by Patricia's mother to alter the temper tantrums?

A good way to remember the three-term contingency is to use the following illustration. We refer to antecedent, behavior, and consequence as the ABCs of behavior:

Antecedent	Behavior	Consequence
A ——————▶	B ——————▶	C

Using the information in the illustration, draw a line from the appropriate term to its meaning:

Behavior (B)	This follows a behavior.
Antecedent (A)	This comes before the behavior.
Consequence (C)	This is observable and measurable; it is also known as a response.

If we implement strategies before a behavior to decrease the likelihood that it will occur, we have implemented antecedent management strategies. Patricia's mother altered the events that preceded Patricia's tantrums by silencing the bell of the telephone. The antecedent influencing the behavior (tantrums) was the noise of the bell. Antecedent strategies can be very effective. If the environment is arranged appropriately, the necessary materials are available, and the means for the child to make his needs and wants known is available, the likelihood of the challenging behavior occurring is lessened.

Basic Questions When Thinking of Antecedent Management

Use the following scenario to learn more about using antecedents to manage behavior:

> Johnny is a 7-year-old boy diagnosed with autism. He has just arrived home from school, and his mother is in the kitchen. Johnny is calmly sitting in his chair in the living room looking through his favorite musical sing-along book. He suddenly begins to bang his fist into his ear with enough force that his mother hears the smacking noise in the kitchen and comes to the living room to see what part of his body he is striking.

How can the preceding situation be evaluated, and what antecedent management strategies can be implemented to help in the future? First, we need to answer the following questions to determine if there is a contributing variable to Johnny's self-injurious behaviors:

1. Is there something in the environment contributing to Johnny's behavior?

2. Is there something medically wrong with him? Does he have an earache?
3. Did someone give him an instruction?
4. What other environmental variables could have contributed to his self-injury?
5. How can knowing the answers to these questions help manage Johnny's self-injury before it occurs again?

These questions provide examples of how to examine antecedent variables that can be contributing to the challenging behavior. Once you have the answers to such questions, you can set up your environment for success. In addition to arranging the environment, other skills can be taught to replace the challenging behaviors:

> Timothy was a 10-year-old boy with autism who was learning basic communication skills. He progressed well in a number of programs involving matching items by their functions, and he could identify the meanings of each of the cards he was to match when they were presented to him individually. His error rate went up considerably when, instead of matching a tool with a tool or an animal with an animal, he was directed to match the tool with the place of use and the animal with its habitat (e.g., "Where do you use the shovel?" and "Where does the fish live?"). His teacher had the impression that Timothy was not thinking before answering, so when she presented the cards from which he was to point out the correct matches, she prevented him from responding by holding the cards in a tray slightly out of his reach. After asking the question, she would say, "Wait and think about your answer." On later trials, she simply said, "Wait." And later she just gestured until he paused for a few seconds. After a few seconds the cards were put in front of him to respond. His error rate decreased considerably because his teacher arranged the environment and gave him the appropriate prompting for him to give correct responses.

Introducing Reinforcement To Reduce Behaviors

Reinforcement increases behaviors that it follows, but as you increase one behavior, you often see a decrease in another. That is how we use reinforcement procedures to *reduce* behavior; we reinforce other behaviors designed to reduce a problem behavior. When a child engages in an appropriate behavior for reinforcement, he or she usually does not simultaneously engage in a problem behavior:

> Jamie talks a great deal, but her topics are very limited. In fact, she speaks primarily about the characters of her favorite Disney movie.

Jamie's parents were pleased that she learned to talk so well, but they were hoping she could begin to communicate more functionally. After defining the behavior of speaking about limited topics and recording a baseline level of that behavior over several days, Jamie's parents decided they would ignore the talk about Disney movies and respond positively when she talked about any other topic. Jamie's problem soon decreased, and she was able to converse more effectively about more topics.

Jamie's parents used reinforcement to increase a behavior that served to also decrease the behavior they were concerned about. The technical term for this is *differential reinforcement of alternative behaviors,* sometimes called DRA, and it is a procedure that is part of most programs designed to reduce behavior. It is sometimes used by itself but is usually used with other procedures, as in the example, in which Jamie's parents ignored the specific problem, talking about a single topic, while implementing the reinforcement program for talk about other topics.

EXERCISE

Refer to the Identifying Behaviors in Need of Reduction section about George engaging in problem behaviors during early language acquisition training. What problem behaviors concerned George's parents? What kind of reinforcement procedures could be used to reduce those problem behaviors?

Other Reinforcement Techniques To Reduce Behavior

As discussed, although reinforcement is used to increase behavior, it can also be used to weaken a problem behavior. There are three common ways to use reinforcement to reduce behavior: (a) reinforce the child for engaging in any behavior other than the target behavior; (b) reinforce the child for not exhibiting the problem behavior for a period of time; and (c) reinforce the child for exhibiting any behavior other than the problem behavior at the end of an interval.

Reinforce the child for engaging in any behavior other than the target behavior. This method of reinforcement was used in Jamie's example to reduce her habit of engaging in narrow topics of conversation. When her parents reinforced topics that did not involve her favorite Disney characters, her range of topics increased and the strength of her narrow topic decreased. Topic creativity resulted in less narrow-topic talking.

It is common to toilet train toddlers by reinforcing them for using the toilet appropriately. That would be another example of DRA. In both the toilet-training example and the example of Jamie's talking, increasing alternative behaviors had the effect of reducing the problem behavior (e.g., narrow conversations and toilet accidents). Occasionally, reinforcement increases both the preferred alternative behavior and the problem behavior. Although that is rare, it is best to choose a behavior to increase that prevents the problem behavior from occurring at the same time.

In some cases, the behavior that is reinforced is *physically* incompatible with the problem behavior. When you reinforce a physically incompatible behavior, it prevents the problem behavior from occurring at that time. When the alternative behavior is incompatible with the problem behavior, the procedure is called "differential reinforcement of an incompatible behavior," or DRI. Mrs. Pott devised a way to reduce hand flapping in her students by reinforcing an incompatible behavior in the following scenario:

> Mrs. Pott teaches a self-contained classroom of middle school students with autism in a regular middle school with typical peers. Some of her students engage in self-stimulatory behavior when transitioning from one activity to another. Ritualistic hand flapping was particularly stigmatizing, and it was thought by the team that students engaging in such behavior would lose access to jobs in the community, a goal anticipated for several of Mrs. Pott's students. To prevent the hand flapping, Mrs. Pott reinforced the students for walking with their hands in their pockets. They could not wave their hands in front of their bodies at the same time. "Hands in pockets" was physically incompatible with hand flapping.

Reinforce the child for not exhibiting the problem behavior for a period of time. This reinforcement procedure is particularly good for situations where the behavior has a distinct beginning and end and does not occur too frequently. This kind of system, called "differential reinforcement of a low rate" (DRL), is a true example of "catching them being good." In other words, you reinforce the child for going longer and longer intervals without exhibiting the problem behavior or exhibiting it as often. It is important to arrange the level of reinforcement to a rate that exceeds the level of the problem behavior. For example, if a child exhibits a problem behavior an average of 10 times per day, the reinforcement rate should be more frequent than that or set at a rate that allows up to 10 responses in a day. In the following example, Peter's teacher chose to use DRL to gradually reduce his problem behaviors:

> Peter was a 9-year-old who played very aggressively with other children. His kicks, hits, shoves, and pushes were counted during recess for 20 minutes, twice each school day. The baseline measures indicated that he exhibited this behavior an average of 10 times per 20-minute recess. The teacher decided to use Peter's token system, which was very effective with other behaviors that he was learning, to address this problem. Checkmarks were exchanged for privileges,

snacks, toys, and free time. Peter's teacher gave him a point and praise for every minute that he did not exhibit the problem of aggressive behaviors. In a short time, he learned to play more gently and without so many aggressive behaviors. Gradually, over a 2-week period, his teacher increased the number of minutes required to receive points without exhibiting the problem behavior.

Reinforce the child for exhibiting any behavior other than the problem behavior at the end of an interval. Especially when the frequency of a problem behavior is very high or it is difficult to continuously observe the child, the best option might be to reinforce the child as frequently as possible when the problem behavior is not occurring. Typically, this reinforcement plan calls for the teacher to observe the child at a given interval for a short time. Reinforcementwouldbegivenifthebehaviorwasnotobservedduringtheshort observation interval. Had the frequency of problem behaviors in Peter's case been much higher or the behaviors occurred for long durations, the sampling method of reinforcement could have been considered.

Communication as an Alternative to Problem Behavior

For many individuals, behavior problems are directly related to their inability to communicate. This relationship represents one of the most important findings in supporting people with behavior disorders. Whereas in the past, behavior disorders were likely to be treated with more restrictive strategies, such as punishment, today we realize that we can often shape communication in children and adults with disabilities to prevent them from resorting to behavior disorders to make their wishes known.

We discussed previously that behavior problems normally have a function for the person exhibiting the behavior. We discover the function or purpose of a behavior by conducting a functional assessment or functional analysis. That information is useful in supporting a person with behavior disorders because we can then help them to communicate that function in a more efficient way than exhibiting problem behaviors (e.g., "Go away!" "I need help," "Can I have one?"). This is called "functional communication training" (FCT).

There are many ways to help people communicate more effectively. Sign language, gesturing, augmentative devices, picture icons, and Picture Exchange Communication System (PECS) cards are all techniques that assist people with communication deficits to communicate more effectively. FCT is a reinforcement procedure developed to replace problem behaviors with communication. There is an inverse relationship between communication skills and problem behaviors. When communication improves and increases, problem behaviors decrease.

Through a functional assessment or analysis, you can determine what function or communicative intent is served by a behavior disorder. Once that function is determined, a corresponding FCT alternative for communicating that need can be established. When functionally analyzed or assessed, most problem behaviors are found to have one of the functions listed in the following table:

Function of the behavior	Communicative intent	FCT alternative
Attention	"Hey! Pay attention to me."	Raise your hand and say, "Excuse me." Tap the person on the shoulder.
Escape	"Go away," "I don't want to do this," "Please, not now."	Give a sign for "Time out, please," or request a break.
Access to a preferred item	"I want that."	Request item or activity using alternative communication strategies.

FCT consists of behavior that is an alternative to the problem behavior. As FCT increases, the problem behavior, seeking the same goal, no longer functions to reach that goal and becomes unnecessary. The FCT behavior must be designed to be more efficient in attaining the goal than the problem behavior. Let's examine the example of Johnny hitting himself in the ear. Johnny was sitting in a chair with his favorite sing-along book and began hitting himself in the ear. What possible variables could have contributed to his behavior, and what functional communication could replace the challenging behavior?

In the next table, possible antecedents of Johnny's behavior are listed in the left column, and potential functional communication training skills are listed in the right column.

Possible antecedent	Functional communication training
Johnny's book stopped playing music.	Teach him to say, "I need help."
Johnny had an earache.	Teach him to exchange a PECS icon for "earache" or "hurt" and "ear."
Johnny's mother told him to come into the kitchen for lunch.	Give him a transition warning, such as "It will be time for lunch in 3 minutes, Johnny," and set a timer to indicate when the 3 minutes is up. You can also teach him to communicate that he would like "1 more minute" when the timer goes off, which gives him more choice and control over the previously troublesome transition.

Review of Reinforcement Procedures To Reduce Behaviors

To reduce behaviors, we recommend the use of one of the reinforcement procedures outlined in this section. Reinforcement procedures have a number of advantages over other procedures used to reduce problem behaviors. For example, reinforcement procedures are accepted by most people as an acceptable way to help a child to learn. Because there is little stigma associated with using positive reinforcement procedures, they can be administered in all settings without concern about embarrassing the child or the adult working with the child. A procedure that is easy to administer consistently in all settings is more likely to be carried out in a way that will promote a successful sustained improvement in behavior.

Reinforcement procedures also have the advantage of promoting better learning across settings and in new situations. For that reason, even if another procedure is used to reduce a problem behavior, a reinforcement procedure is also recommended. After all, it is usually considered best to teach an appropriate behavior to take the place of a problem behavior. The reinforcing procedures we have described serve that function.

EXERCISES

Now you are ready to practice designing programs that use reinforcement to reduce behaviors:

1. On a piece of paper, list five problem behaviors that concern you, define each behavior, choose a method of measurement, and identify a preferred behavior that is potentially incompatible with the problem behavior. Share your answers with another person doing the same exercise. Did you both answer the questions of who, what, how, when, and where in your definitions? Did you agree that your preferred behaviors were potentially incompatible?

2. Observe one of the problem behaviors you listed in at least two settings. Record the behavior in accordance with your definition, and note the events preceding and following the behavior. Derive the function of the behavior and a potential form of functional communication that could replace the problem behavior. Again, share your findings with a colleague or supervisor. Did your colleague agree with you? If not, more baseline observations with functional assessment may be necessary; but if you have agreement, you can begin to support the child with a reinforcement procedure with or without FCT. *Remember to always use a reinforcement procedure in combination with any other reduction procedures used.*

Interrupting the Consequences That Maintain Behavior

Because unwanted behavior is shaped and maintained by the events that come after it, another way to reduce behavior involves identifying the consequences maintaining the behavior and interrupting or removing them. In most cases, reinforcement that is not intended is occurring after a problem behavior. In this section we will discuss how to identify that reinforcing consequence and withhold it after the problem behavior. This process is technically called "extinction," and it is very effective in reducing behaviors controlled by the events coming after them.

Problem behaviors are often followed by the attention of others in the child's environment. In other cases, giving the child what he or she wants may inadvertently strengthen a problem behavior. For those scenarios we often use *planned ignoring* to prevent the child from receiving attention or a tangible reinforcement for a problem behavior. Ironically, those consequences may have developed to calm the child. Many parents give children what they want, even if their "request" comes in the form of a problem behavior.

Return to the example of Jamie described earlier in this chapter and answer the following questions:

1. When Jamie began to talk about Disney characters in excess, what were the probable consequences of that behavior?
2. How was planned ignoring accomplished with Jamie?

As we have said, behaviors are often controlled by their consequences. When a child exhibits a problem behavior, we are particularly interested in the consequences of that behavior and attempt to determine what events follow it. Problem behaviors are often followed by the attention of others, as mentioned. For example, when a parent is in the checkout line of the grocery store busily attending to the groceries, a child's attempt to reach out and grab an attractive candy bar beside the cash register is likely to be met with a scolding or directive by the parent. For the child whose parent has not spoken to her for a few minutes, that attention is likely to be a powerful consequence that reinforces the child's behavior.

In an alternative scenario, the parent, anxious to proceed with the shopping and get home, gives the candy to the child. In that case, the child does not receive much attention for attempting to get the candy bar but actually receives the desired candy. That is an important *tangible* consequence, which also increases the likelihood that, under similar conditions, the child will exhibit the same behavior.

Attention and tangible rewards are not the only consequences that maintain problem behaviors; other events may be involved as well. For example, self-stimulatory behaviors such as the hand flapping exhibited by Mrs. Pott's students may not be affected by changes in one's attention to the behavior. Many behaviors of that kind are maintained automatically by the visual, auditory, or other stimulation derived from the behavior.

Because consequences such as attention, tangible items, and automatic reinforcement serve to strengthen and maintain problem behaviors, we naturally attempt to prevent those consequences. Many of the consequences that maintain problem behaviors are important for the child, however. We would never advocate removing attention from a child permanently, because children need our attention to learn. We advocate removing or withholding attention only after problem behaviors. When a consequence that strengthens a problem behavior is removed or withheld after the problem behavior, it also can be provided for an appropriate alternative behavior. For example, if a problem behavior has consistently been followed with attention, the adults in the child's home and classroom could be careful to provide positive attention for periods of time without the problem behavior or when an alternative to the problem behavior occurs, while withholding attention after the problem behavior. During difficult tasks, some children exhibit problem behaviors that will facilitate their escape from or avoidance of the task. When escape opportunities are found to consistently follow a problem behavior, a program may be initiated to give the student a break after completing only a small portion of the unpleasant task. In that way, escape from the task is used to reinforce completion of the task, and gradually the portion of the task required for a break is increased.

Most procedures that interrupt consequences also use reinforcement of other behaviors to increase their therapeutic effects. Reinforcing other behaviors helps to promote sustained changes and can decrease the negative side effects associated with the removal of reinforcing consequences that have previously been available. The interruption of instrumental consequences that influence a problem behavior can have excellent results that maintain nicely, but in some cases the problem behavior may get worse before it gets better. Professionals refer to this common phenomenon as an *extinction burst.* Those supporting a child for whom reinforcers are being withheld should be prepared to tolerate some increases in the problem behavior before it decreases.

Time-Out

Using time-out can often produce effects similar to those produced by successful planned ignoring and other forms of extinction. Time-out or time-out from positive reinforcement removes the person exhibiting the behavior from the reinforcement for a period of time. First rigorously tested in the 1960s, time-out has become a part of the American culture, although it often is not implemented correctly. Its early applications involved placing a child in a time-out room after the child exhibited a problem behavior. Concerns arising out of placing children alone in rooms have been raised over the years, so today most time-out applications involve milder forms of the procedure. For example, following disruptive behavior in a classroom setting, some teachers ask the child to sit away from the ongoing activity for a period of time. This is called a "nonexclusionary time-out" because the child is not actually removed from the environment in which reinforcement is accessible.

Time-In

Crucial to the success of a time-out procedure is an enriched "time-in." For example, if the ongoing activity from which the child is removed is reinforcing, time-out will have a greater likelihood of success. If, on the other hand, a child is exhibiting a problem behavior to escape a task or activity, time-out would not be recommended because it would satisfy the child's goal of escaping. By the same token, if the child preferred time alone to engage in some solitary behavior such as self-stimulatory behavior, time-out could become a reinforcing event leading to increased problem behaviors. When used correctly under the right conditions, time-out can be very effective and help the child to learn more appropriate behaviors. In some cases, the time-in environment is made more reinforcing by providing *noncontingent reinforcement,* in which adults intentionally provide praise or other reinforcers on a schedule, regardless of the behaviors being exhibited. If a child has been seeking attention by exhibiting a problem behavior and family and teachers provide him or her with lots of attention throughout the day, it becomes unnecessary for the child to exhibit the problem behavior.

Contingent Reinforcement Loss

A third form of reinforcement manipulation used to reduce behaviors is *contingent reinforcement loss.* This procedure involves removing an amount of reinforcement following a problem behavior. The loss may involve money (as in the fine you get for speeding in your vehicle), tokens, or other reinforcers held or consumed slowly. It is important for this procedure to be used in conjunction with a reinforcement system for appropriate behavior, and it is usually advised that the rate of reinforcers given should be significantly higher than the rate of reinforcement loss. The following description illustrates a program that uses contingent reinforcement loss with time-out:

> Victor had attended a self-contained classroom in his local middle school for 2 years when his IEP team began to focus on developing his independence in completing tasks and his acquisition of marketable vocational skills to attain employment in the community. Victor had made significant progress academically with the help of a point system in which good work completed accurately and on time earned him points to spend on activities of his choosing.
> As he was learning vocational skills, it became apparent that he engaged in some behaviors that could be offensive to people in

the community. For example, he would indiscreetly adjust his underwear in an inappropriate manner and burp loudly without any apparent concern or remorse. His team was concerned that his access to jobs would be limited if he continued to exhibit these problem behaviors.

After defining the behaviors, obtaining good reliability of their measures, and obtaining a baseline, his treatment team approved the use of a point fine for exhibiting the problem behaviors. It was explained to Victor before the implementation of the procedure that the behaviors would limit his job prospects and that he would be more welcome at job sites if he was able to control the behaviors, which some people would find offensive. The point fine was just the reminder Victor needed to learn to exhibit the problem behaviors less frequently or in a private location, such as the bathroom. His behavior improved nicely over the next few weeks during the periods of time when he was earning points. At home and during the weekends and during times when he was spending his points on a favorite activity, the offensive behaviors were still exhibited. In response to this, his team consulted with Victor and recommended that he would have to take a brief time-out from his preferred activity if he engaged in offensive behavior. Typically, this was accomplished by prompting Victor to leave his activity and go to the bathroom for a minute until he could return without any burping or clothing adjustments.

That combination of contingent reinforcement loss and time-out during reinforcing activities proved to be very effective for Victor. He also really enjoyed the praise and attention of his staff and parents, but he was most happy when he got his first job, at a local restaurant for a good hourly wage.

EXERCISES

1. Match the procedure to the description:

   Extinction   Removes an amount of reinforcement from the child.

   Time-out   Withholds reinforcement from the child following a problem behavior.

   Contingent   Removes child from the reinforcer
   reinforcement loss   for a specified period of time.

2. Go back to the description of Emily in the Identifying Behaviors in Need of Reduction section of this booklet and define her problem behavior.

3. Describe how you might interrupt, withhold, or remove the reinforcing consequences maintaining Emily's behavior.

4. When first described, autism was thought to be the result of parents not caring for their children in a loving manner. Mothers of children with autism were referred to as "refrigerator mothers," and recommendations revolved around finding a way for the parents to become warmer and more loving. With this misunderstanding, recommendations often revolved around loving the children more and comforting them when problem behaviors occurred. What would you expect to be the outcome of this kind of procedure? If the behavior increased with this procedure, what would you think was maintaining the problem behaviors?

Introducing Events That Discourage Behavior

The fourth category of methods to reduce problem behavior includes procedures that are specifically designed and implemented to reduce a behavior. When thinking about reducing behaviors, most people first think of events like scolding, spanking, traffic fines, and events of that kind. The term *punishment* is often used when talking about reducing behavior. Our options for actively reducing behaviors are broad, but before reviewing all of them, it would be useful to discuss and define *punishment* here, as well as the role it may play in supporting children.

Punishment

Behavior analysis defines punishment based on its effects on the behavior it follows. That is, punishment would be something that decreases behavior that it follows. Although spanking would serve as a punisher, many other events could meet this definition of punishment as well. For example, if a student volunteers an answer to a question in class that is incorrect, the teacher will likely tell the student about the error. If the student responded to that feedback by not answering that question the same way again, the teacher's feedback would meet the behavior analysis definition of punishment.

Much of the literature about punishment, oddly, is related to harsh consequences that involve painful, noxious, or extremely unpleasant events, even though childcare professionals rarely recommend severe procedures of that kind. It is also interesting that much of the literature about punishment directed at parents indicates that it does not work. When considering punishment from the perspective of applied behavior analysis, we need to reevaluate our understanding. By accepted behavioral definitions, an event would not be punishment if it did not decrease a behavior it followed. There

35

are other factors leading people away from using punishment, but punishment can work and may sometimes be the best option for a problem behavior.

Our definition of punishment, therefore, is based on what happens to the behavior it follows. For example, correcting a student's incorrect answers would not normally be considered a punishment procedure. Nevertheless, feedback would be considered a viable and acceptable method of reducing incorrect answers and would meet the behavioral definition of punishment.

Most behavior analysts list time-out and contingent reinforcement loss, both described previously, as punishment procedures. Those methods also involve procedures that reduce behaviors they follow. So punishment, when viewed by its effect on behavior, can include procedures that would be especially useful in supporting children with severe problem behaviors.

Undoubtedly, the objections to punishment result from the warranted concerns around harsh consequences that could cause more harm than good for the recipient. For example, a student providing an incorrect answer may come no closer to determining the correct answer if he or she is told only that he or she is wrong. Of more use would be information that would enable the student to identify and recall the correct answer. For that reason, we recommend that children with behavior disorders be provided with reinforcers and other encouraging support to learn the correct behavior to replace a problem response.

Teachers, parents, and other adults who are caretakers for a child with behavior disorders can effectively and independently implement many of the procedures described in this book. When using one of the procedures included in the behavioral definition of punishment, the support of a professional with extensive experience is advised. Even simple and acceptable forms of punishment have potential pitfalls, as we have described. In addition, directly reducing a problem behavior with a punishment procedure requires coordination of all who come in contact with the child, as well as the approval of the child's parent or guardian.

Effort

The final procedures useful in reducing problem behaviors involve the use of effort. Effort procedures require some activity from the child. Effort can be used as a consequence, such as having a child correct an error (contingent effort), or it can be used as an antecedent (response requirement).

Contingent effort. Many forms of effort call for the child to change his or her behavior immediately following a problem behavior. This may be called "correction, interruption, or redirection."

Correction is demonstrated in the following example:

Andrew destroyed property when he became upset. If he were seated at his desk in school, he would sometimes kick the desk across the room, risking injury to others in the room. On other occasions, in a temper tantrum, he would throw chairs or books or rip papers off the bulletin board. After much consideration and a period of baseline observations, his team decided that he would have to repair all the destruction he caused in his environment. If he displaced furniture, he would have to set it back in place; if he destroyed the bulletin board, he would have to replace all the items the way they were.

Interruption and redirection are demonstrated in this example:

Allen was a hand flapper. After his teachers gathered baseline measures, they decided that every time he flapped his hands while he was away from his desk, he would be directed to put his hands in his pockets. If he flapped them while engaging in a task, his problem behavior would be interrupted and he would be directed to complete the task. A reinforcement procedure was included, according to which Allen would be praised for stopping the flapping and engaging in the alternative behaviors.

Other forms of effort may involve prompting the child to engage in a behavior that goes beyond correction, interruption, or redirection. In some cases, the effort is a form of exercise or a task to put the environment into a condition that exceeds correction. For example, for property destruction, if Andrew was required not only to correct the disruption made to the environment but also to mop the floors and wash the walls, the effort would be called "overcorrection." If he was required to run a lap every time he destroyed property, that would be called "contingent exercise." Effort may also come in the form of practicing an appropriate response. A common method of reducing toilet accidents, called "positive practice," involves going from the place of the toilet accident to the bathroom several times. These extended forms of effort have been successfully implemented and validated and may be another option for use with children with problem behaviors.

Although *contingent effort* is a mild form of aversive control, it can nevertheless be misused. The form of effort used as a consequence should have five attributes: (a) the task should be easily prompted with a minimum of physical guidance; (b) the task should comprise behaviors that are frequently exhibited by the child; (c) the task should be unobtrusive so it can be carried out in all settings; (d) the task should not inflict any unnecessary strain on the child; and (e) each performance of the task should be of relatively short duration.

As with all procedures of this kind, contingent effort may result in an increase in escape and avoidance behaviors such as whining, crying, or even aggression. It should always be paired with a reinforcement procedure to ensure that the child is encouraged to exhibit a more appropriate form of behavior in place of the problem behavior being reduced. It is particularly important to determine the functions of problem behaviors before implementing any procedure, particularly one like contingent effort, which may not be effective with behaviors exhibited for attention or to escape tasks.

Response requirement. The final method of using effort to reduce behavior involves making it more difficult to exhibit the target behavior. "Response requirement," as it is called, has been shown to be effective in reducing but not eliminating behavior. In the scenario about Timothy, he was asked a question but not allowed to respond for a few seconds. He was required to sit quietly. Slowing down his responses improved his accuracy. In this case, sitting quietly before responding was response requirement.

Response requirement can be very helpful in slowing behaviors like eating and preventing preschoolers from shifting tasks before completing them. Building intermediate behaviors such as putting down utensils, wiping one's mouth with a napkin, and swallowing before taking the next bite reduces dangerous high-rate eating. Preschoolers may be required to complete one task before switching to another or to ask permission before leaving their desk. Both measures encourage children to exhibit a behavior at an acceptable low rate.

EXERCISES

1. Ricardo was toilet trained during the day but was still wetting his bed. It was his mother's impression that his problem was related to the fact that Ricardo slept so soundly; he was not able to wake up when he had to go to the bathroom. What form of contingent exercise might help Ricardo learn to get himself to the bathroom even if he was very sleepy?
2. Go back to the account about Brianna in the What Controls Problem Behavior section of this booklet. What was the problem behavior targeted for reduction?
3. How was response requirement used to reduce Brianna's problem behavior?

Step Four: Evaluating and Maintaining Change

Once you have successfully defined the challenging behavior, assessed it, and determined a treatment option, how do you evaluate whether your treatment is effective? Anecdotally, it may appear that the behavior is improving or not, but impressions are not always the same as facts. For example, the behavior may have been improving before your procedure was introduced, or changes in the behavior may have been so subtle that they were hard to detect. The most effective way to evaluate change is to have a visual representation of the behavior in a graph. This will allow you to illustrate what the behavior looked like prior to your intervention and following the implementation of your intervention.

A graph will indicate time across the horizontal axis and strength of the behavior on the vertical axis. For example, if you use frequency recording, you would place the number of times the behavior occurred on the vertical axis and perhaps days on the horizontal axis. A description of a program for Barry's aggressive behavior and a graph of his performance follows:

> Barry's teacher and parents decided it was necessary to intervene with his hitting behavior because it was causing him to stay out of special programs at school and his siblings did not like to interact with him at home. His parents and teacher began by taking baseline data. Baseline indicated that Barry was hitting up to 25 times per day. During the baseline data collection, they also conducted a functional assessment in which they took data on what was happening before the hitting and what occurred after. According to the data, Barry was hitting his teacher, peers, and family members when they could not quickly determine what he was asking of them. Based upon these results, the family and teacher decided to teach Barry how to use a communication system to make his needs and wants better known. This intervention helped greatly in reducing his hitting. The few instances in which he hit after the communication was implemented occurred when the teacher was out of the classroom and his communication system was not used properly. It was decided to graph data from both home and school to see if the introduction of the communication system also worked at home. The data in Figure 3 suggest the intervention was successful in both settings.

According to the graph in Figure 3, the intervention chosen for Barry was successful because it dropped the number of hits per day to an acceptable number for both his family and his teacher. It is important to represent your data graphically so that you have a visual representation of whether the intervention is working. Practice your graphing skill using the information in the following scenario:

> Lauren was an 8-year-old girl diagnosed with mild mental retardation who attended a multihandicapped classroom with five other students with a variety of developmental disabilities. She often exhibited inappropriate vocalizations during school. These were loud, belch-like noises that were loud enough to disrupt class. Other

students gave her attention for this behavior and had been seen giggling and laughing with Lauren following her belches.

The teacher decided to establish a rule for the class for belching and inappropriate laughter after belching. A system was set up in which students earned extra time in the activities or recess portions of the day if there were no belches or inappropriate laughing or fewer belches and laughter than were recorded the day before. Use the data that follow to chart the behavior on the graph provided; then answer the questions about the data.

Days	Number of Belches
Before Intervention	
1	15
2	16
3	15
4	13
5	12
6	17
After Intervention	
7	20
8	15
9	4
10	3
11	2
12	0

EXERCISES

1. Graph the first 6 days of behavior according to numbers listed.
2. Connect the data path.
3. Label the first 6 days of data as "Baseline."
4. Draw a vertical line to separate baseline data from data collected following the intervention.
5. Graph the last 6 days of data and connect the data points.
6. How should these data be labeled?

If your graph looks like the one in Figure 4, well done! Was the intervention successful? What happened to the number of belches after planned ignoring was introduced?

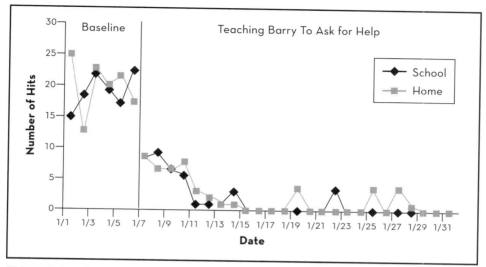

FIGURE 3. The number of times Barry hit others each day. Data compiled in Barry's school and home are graphed separately. During baseline, no changes were made in the daily routine for Barry. After 7 days, Barry was provided with a functional communication system through which he could more clearly make his needs and wants known. The data suggest that with the improved communication system, Barry's hits decreased significantly.

As is often the case, Lauren's problem behavior actually increased before it decreased with planned ignoring. Luckily, her teacher and parents were familiar with extinction bursts before they started the ignoring program.

Step Five: Maintaining Changes Across Environments

Reducing serious problem behaviors is helpful only if the improved rate of behavior can be maintained. This concept is called "maintenance." It is also important for the child to exhibit the improved behavior in different settings and with different people. This concept is called *generalization.* If Johnny exhibits the low rate of self-injury when he is with his favorite teacher but exhibits higher rates at home or with other staff, that is not considered a successful change in behavior.

Depending on the method used to reduce behavior, maintaining the improved rate of behavior and ensuring that the improvement is exhibited in all settings can present a challenge. Behavior changes that occur as a

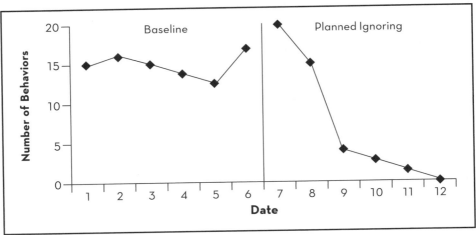

FIGURE 4. The correct depiction of data described in the previous exercise and collected on Lauren's belches each school day. During baseline, belches were recorded without any specific contingencies. During planned ignoring, the other students were informed about the behavior and instructed not to laugh or giggle when Lauren exhibited the inappropriate vocalizations. In addition, the class was allowed extra time for recess or in an activity of their choosing for decreases in Lauren's belches and reactions from the other students. Student reactions were immediately eliminated with the introduction of the planned ignoring procedure. Lauren's belches gradually decreased over the observation period and were eliminated on the sixth day of the ignoring program.

result of reinforcement can usually be maintained more easily than changes accomplished through other procedures, such as punishment. Ironically, if a behavior is increasing in strength, missing an opportunity to reinforce the alternative behavior can actually strengthen the behavior. Remember the extinction burst? If a behavior being suppressed with one of the other procedures, such as contingent effort or contingent reinforcement loss, is exhibited without the suppressive consequence, it can be strengthened, and your intervention can be weakened.

In order for the improved lower rates of behavior to be maintained, you need to plan for maintenance and generalization from the beginning. There are four methods of promoting successful maintenance and generalization:

1. *Reinforce an appropriate alternative behavior.* As we have discussed, reinforcing an alternative behavior may cause the frequency or level of the problem behavior to decrease. In many instances, differential reinforcement of alternative behavior can be used without other procedures to reduce behavior to acceptable levels. For example, the scenario about Jimmy's ag-

gressive behavior during playtime (see the Introduction to Applied Behavior Analysis section in this booklet) illustrated a successful program in which points were given to Jimmy for periods of time with no sharing problems. Positive reinforcement procedures have lasting effects and generalize well. Many suppressive procedures do not generalize as well. For example, if a child exhibits a behavior for attention, a time-out from attention may be used following each inappropriate response. It would be necessary to supplement the time-out with reinforcement (e.g., providing attention for behavior that is incompatible with the problem behavior). By using one of the reinforcement procedures (e.g., one of the differential reinforcement procedures or functional communication training), you will have an easier time attaining maintenance and generalization.

2. *Use procedures that are the most natural.* Procedures should be appropriate to the settings in which they will be used. Implementing a simple procedure is preferred to using one that is complicated and requires a lot of effort from the people implementing it to ensure that it is used across settings and with different people. It is essential that the procedure chosen can be implemented in the school, at home, at Grandma's house, and in the park during a play date, for example.

3. *Use the procedure across all settings.* Make sure you use a procedure that can be implemented in all settings and with all the people the individual works and lives with. If you use a procedure in the school but not in the home, generalization will not occur. Sometimes you might choose a weaker procedure because it can more realistically be implemented in all settings. For example, you might choose reinforcement of other behaviors instead of a time-out because families may not always be able to complete the time-out procedure. It is important to identify how the procedure will be carried out in all settings. Ensuring that whatever procedure is used is implemented in all settings will promote long-lasting change.

4. *Once you have reached an acceptable level of the problem behavior, fade the treatment procedure.* If a problem behavior is completely eliminated, the procedure will be faded automatically. In many cases, however, the problem behavior can be acceptably reduced to lower levels, requiring a plan to fade the reduction procedure in a way that will preserve the improved level of the behavior. For example, in the beginning of a reinforcement procedure, you may present an edible for every minute of appropriate behavior or non-occurrence of the problem behavior. As the child becomes successful with the 1-minute DRL, you gradually shift the reinforcement to every 90 seconds, then every 2 minutes, and so on. Eventually, you would want to fade the delivery of the edible to a more natural schedule, such as midmorning snack time, after lunch, and then afternoon snack. The following scenario illustrates how Justin's program was faded:

Justin is a 10-year-old boy who has been diagnosed with autism and exhibits high rates of inappropriate touching of others. He will often try to gain others' attention by touching them on their private areas (e.g., touching women in their genital area and then looking for their reaction) or pulling their hair. Justin has started a new school, and his teachers and family have defined these behaviors in preparation for reduction. On Justin's first day, he is paired with a one-to-one staff person, and noncontingent praise is delivered throughout the day. If inappropriate touching occurs, it is ignored. This noncontingent reinforcement is eventually faded to a DRL in which he receives a token every minute toward playing a game with his favorite teacher.

See if you can answer the following questions for the preceding example:

1. What is the next step to fade the DRL for Justin?
2. Justin has been successful with his DRL and has decreased his inappropriate touching in school, but he still pulls his sister's hair and touches his mom inappropriately. What could you do to promote generalization to the home environment?
3. What is an alternative behavior you could teach Justin to gain attention, rather than inappropriately touching others?

Conclusion

Ifa behavior significantly impedes a person's ability to function on his or her own or to the benefit of society, it is deemed a problem behavior and must be eliminated or reduced. We have reviewed a number of procedures used to support children in this process, and we have given examples of a variety of problem behaviors in a variety of settings. Effective management of problem behaviors involves more than simply reducing the problem behavior. Full support of the child with problem behavior must be viewed as an educational process in which a child reduces problem behavior while developing and increasing functional skills.

We have described the process of working to reduce problem behaviors with several important steps:

1. The behavior must truly be a problem for the child. It must be hindering the child's abilities to progress to his or her potential and access as much in life as possible. The decision to reduce a child's behavior should be made by all the people involved with and responsible for his or her development.
2. The behavior must be carefully defined.
3. The behavior must be measured to determine its baseline level. The strength and trend of the behavior should be determined by graphing the measures obtained by observation.
4. The environmental events influencing the behavior both before and after it is exhibited must be assessed and understood. The selection of a procedure to reduce a problem behavior must be chosen with full understanding of its advantages and limitations. If the procedure or one similar to it has been used successfully with the child in the past, one may expect similar success in the future. The procedure selected should be the least intrusive procedure likely to succeed in reducing the problem behavior in all settings.
5. The change in behavior relative to baseline should be analyzed with the help of graphed data.
6. Positive reinforcement and other behavior acquisition procedures must be in place to promote sustained improvements in behavior in all settings. Any active procedures in place to reduce

behaviors should be faded to levels that are available to other children.

In the preceding chapter, you were asked to describe a problem behavior exhibited by a person you know. Summarize a plan to help support that person through the process of reducing his or her problem behavior by answering the following questions:

1. How would you define the behavior?
    a. Who exhibits the problem behavior?
    b. What is the behavior?
    c. How will you measure it?
    d. When will you measure it?
    e. Where will you measure it?
    f. Who will test the measurement reliability?
2. What specific procedures will you use to reduce the behavior?
3. Where will those procedures be carried out?
4. Who will carry out those procedures?
5. How will you plan for maintenance and generalization of the improved behavior?
6. How will you determine whether the program is effective?

References

Baer, D. M., Wolf, M., & Risley, T. R. (1968). Current dimensions of applied behavior analysis. *Journal of Applied Behavior Analysis, 1,* 91–97.

Bailey, J. S., & Burch, M. R. (2002). *Research methods in applied behavior analysis.* Thousand Oaks, CA: Sage.

Cooper, J. O., Heron, T. E., & Heward, W. L. (1987). *Applied behavior analysis.* Columbus, OH: Merrill.

Lovaas, O. I. (2003). *Teaching individuals with developmental delays: Basic intervention.* Austin, TX: PRO-ED.

Luce, S. C., & Christian, W. P. (1981). *How to reduce autistic and severely maladaptive behaviors.* Austin, TX: PRO-ED.

Maurice, C., Green, G., & Luce, S. C. (Eds.). (1996). *Behavioral intervention for the young child with autism: A manual for parents and professionals.* Austin, TX: PRO-ED.

Miltenberger, R. G. (2001). *Behavior modification: Principles and procedures* (2nd ed.). Belmont, CA: Wadsworth/Thomson.

Sidman, M. (1966). *Tactics of scientific research: Evaluating experimental data in psychology.* Oxford, England: Basic Books.

Sulzer-Azaroff, B., & Mayer, G. R. (1991). *Behavior analysis for lasting change.* New York: Holt, Rinehart & Winston.

About the Editor and Authors

Richard L. Simpson is professor of special education at the University of Kansas. He currently directs several federally supported projects to prepare teachers and leadership professionals for careers with children and youth with autism spectrum disorders. Simpson has also worked as a teacher of students with disabilities, a psychologist, and an administrator of several programs for students with autism. He is the former editor of the professional journal *Focus on Autism and Other Developmental Disabilities* (published by PRO-ED) and the author of numerous books and articles on autism spectrum disorders.

Stephen C. Luce, PhD, a licensed psychologist and board-certified behavior analyst, is the vice president for clinical programs, training, and research of Melmark, a comprehensive human service agency serving adults and children with neurological and developmental disorders, including mental retardation, autism, and acquired brain injuries. Luce received his doctorate in 1979 in developmental and child psychology from the University of Kansas. He also holds a master's degree in education from the Division of Exceptional Children at the University of Georgia and an AB degree in psychology from Marietta College in Ohio. Luce has spent much of his career as a teacher and psychologist working with children with developmental disorders and behavioral disorders. He is the author of numerous articles, chapters, and monographs published in professional journals and books. His most popular book at this time is *Behavioral Intervention for the Young Child with Autism: A Manual for Parents and Professionals,* which he edited with Dr. Catherine Maurice and Dr. Gina Green.

Angela F. Smith, MA, a board-certified behavior analyst, is the clinical director of children's programming at Melmark, based in Berwyn, Pennsylvania. Smith received her master's degree in applied behavior analysis from Penn State University in Harrisburg. She was previously an in-home intensive behavior therapist for young children with autism based in Columbus, Ohio, and a psychometrician at Children's Hospital in Columbus. She completed internships at the Hershey Medical Center Feeding Clinic, Penn State University, and Melmark. She has served as the editorial assistant for the journal *Behavioral Interventions* and was the secretary and program chair for the Pennsylvania Association of Behavior Analysis. Her peer-reviewed publications include work she has done in the assessment and treatment of sleep problems, feeding problems, and other problem behaviors in children with autism.

Both authors can be reached at Melmark, 2600 Wayland Road, Berwyn, PA 19312, or through the Melmark Web site (www.melmark.org). The authors wish to thank their colleagues and the leadership of Melmark for their support in writing this manuscript, particularly Dr. Joanne Gillis-Donovan, PhD, RN, chief executive of Melmark. They also acknowledge Walter P. Christian, PhD, who co-authored the first version of this material. Correspondence about this booklet can be directed to Dr. Luce.